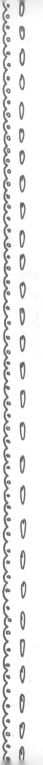

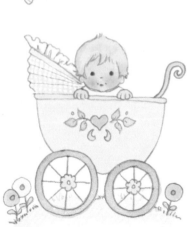

A
Baby
Girl...
Congratulations!

The C.R. Gibson Company · Norwalk, Connecticut

Congratulations on your
new baby girl!

From the top of her head to her tiny toes, this little bundle of loveliness will bless your lives with joy and delight.

And may your
hearts be filled with the
happiness of bringing a
new human being into
the universe — to laugh,
to love, to know the
wonder of life and the
beauty of the world we
live in!

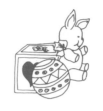

There are booties
and bottles
everywhere,

A feeling of
happiness in
the air,

Talcum and
blankets and
a teddy bear.

But who cares if
things are
in disarray...

What a wonderful
happening
they convey—

YOU'RE BRINGING
YOUR BABY
GIRL HOME
TODAY!

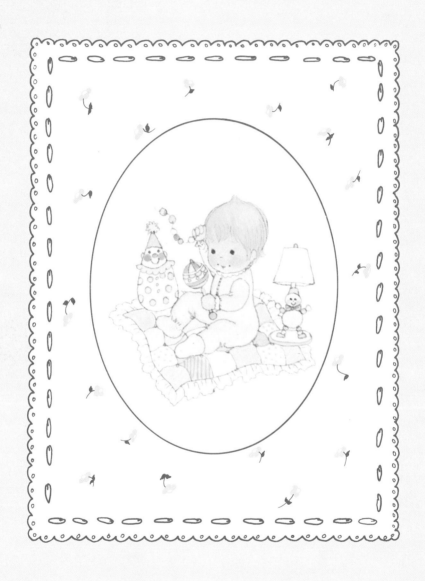

Marvel of all marvels —
a baby girl! Tiny
mouth, shining eyes,
a wisp of hair — so
perfect, so endearing.
Small miracle fresh
from heaven, life's
greatest gift, God's
Masterpiece!

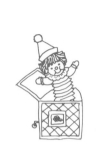

What are you
   thinking of,

Little one,

Whose life on
   this earth

Has just begun?

Your mind is
    so fresh

And there's
    so much
    to know,

So many
    tomorrows—

So much
    time to grow.

The grown-ups
    love to watch her,
And they join in
    with her coos.
She's the center
    of attraction,
Always getting
    rave reviews!

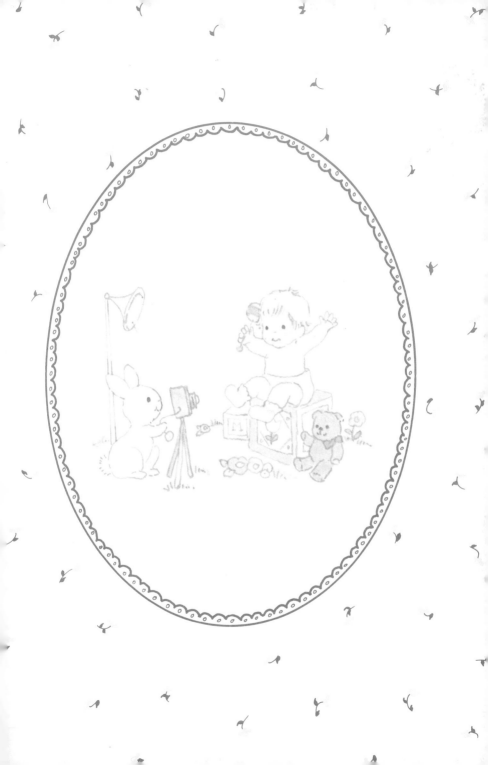

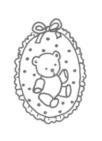

When a little
girl

Discovers her toes,

She laughs and
brings them

Right up to
her nose...

Playing with
them

Prompts a squeal
of delight —

Such fun to
wiggle,

So delicious to
bite!

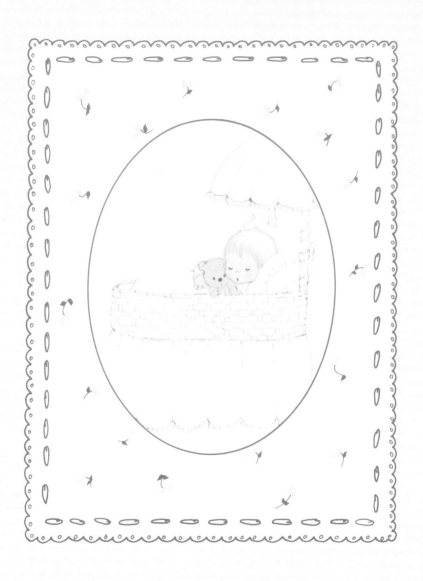

How soul-satisfying it is to hold your baby girl close to your heart! So warm, so soft, sweet and cuddly... A little wonder! An expression of your love!

In the sparkling
eyes of a
baby girl

Heaven and
angels shine,

A veritable
miracle —

A perfect God-
design!

She looks into
the mirror

And sees
a little elf.

Does she think
it's another
baby,

Or does she
realize it's
herself?

She starts with a bottle,
but very soon
your baby is learning
to handle a spoon...
Sometimes the spoon
doesn't quite find
her mouth —
Landing a bit to the
north, west or
south!

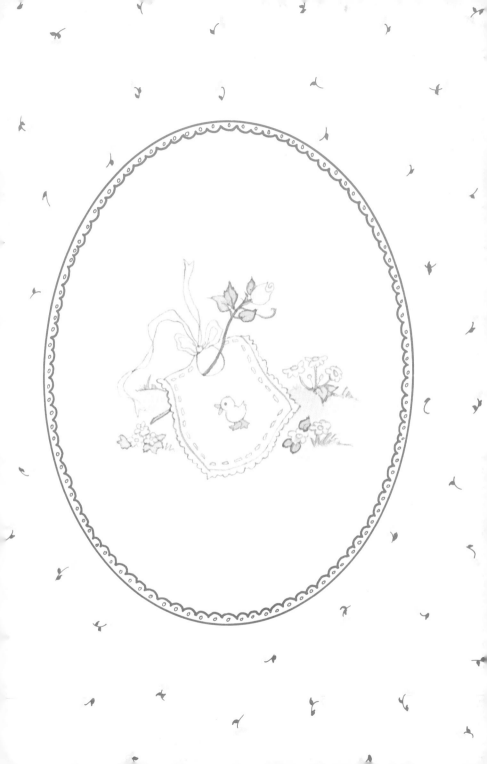

Asleep in her crib, dwarfed even by her tiny teddy bear, not a toddling temptress yet, she's yours now.

As your dreams for
her multiply, your love
for her will grow... yet
never will you forget
the picture of that
small, sweet sleeping
face.

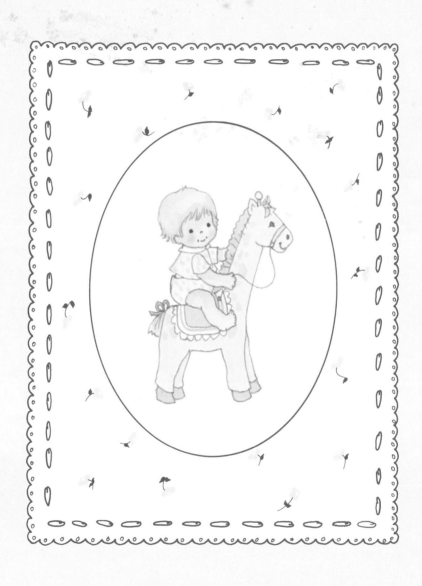

A little girl is part
elf and part angel.
She has an innocent
smile on her face
and, at the same
time, a twinkle in
her eye....

Very early she wraps
her parents around her
finger. And how could
they resist her!

She is a product of
their love, fulfillment of
their dreams. She has
a woman's magic and
charm, a little girl's
enchantment and vision!

The merriest Christmas ever... when joyous parents first play Santa Claus for their baby girl. How her eyes dance in the tree lights as she reaches for the tinsel and bright ornaments!

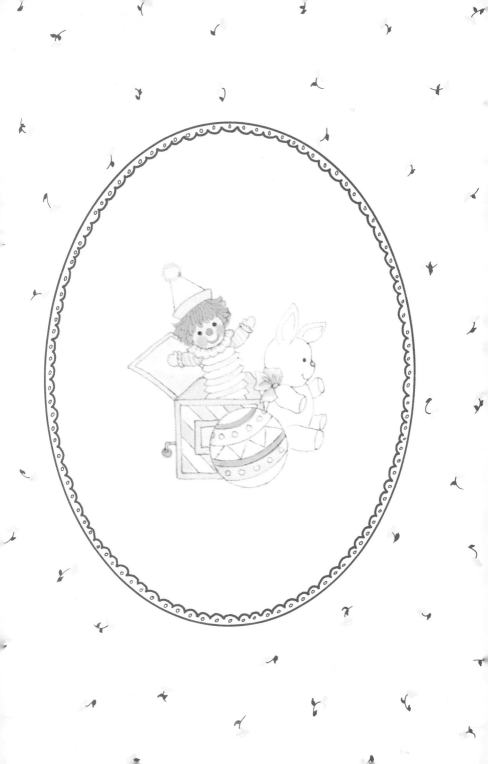

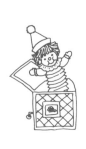

She tries her
best

To stay awake.

(She might miss
something

If she takes
a break!)

But finally
the Sandman

Takes over her
keeping —

So, tiptoe
around her...

Shhhh! She
is sleeping!

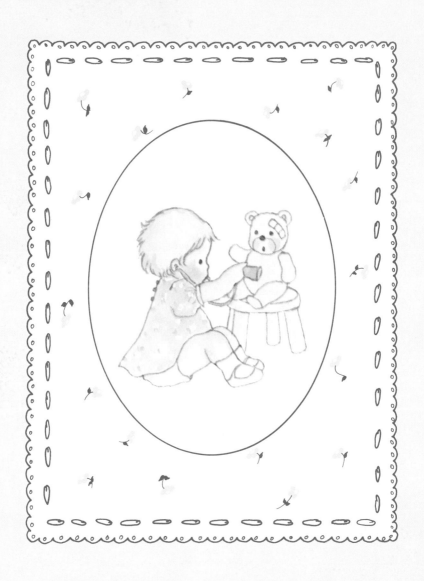

Her first word? Maybe
    Dada or Mama—
Whatever she says,
    it's a thrill!
It's something that
    <u>she</u> won't remember—
But her parents most
    certainly will!

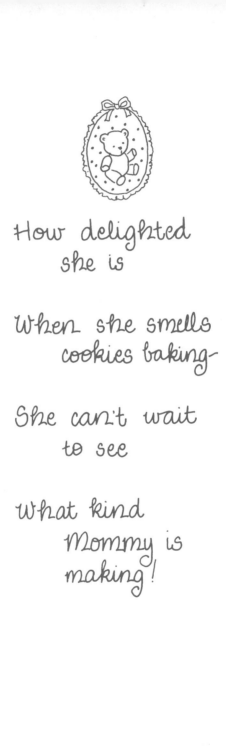

How delighted
she is

When she smells
cookies baking-

She can't wait
to see

What kind
Mommy is
making!

She's confident
she'll be

Allotted her
share,

And if she's
_real_ good —

Maybe even
a spare!

A treat for your
baby
When she's just a
bit older
Will be watching
the world
From Daddy's strong
shoulder!

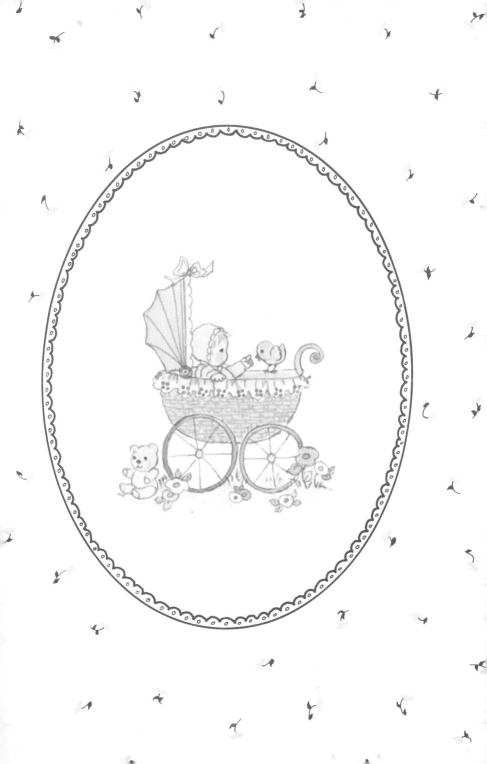

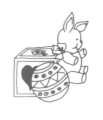

She's learning
to walk,

And it won't
be long now

(Though she
falls pretty
often)

Until she
knows how.

She won't
    cry when
    she falls

For she's done
    it before —

After all,
    when she
    falls,

It's not far
    to the floor!

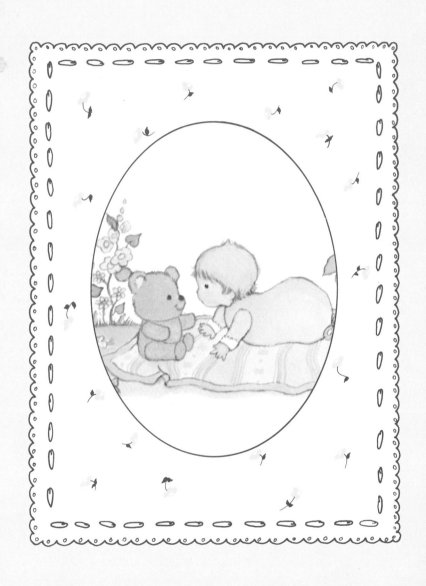

A little girl...
        Bubbling laughter,
tousled hair, a creature full
of bright expectations, dreams
intact, hopes heart-high.
Look at her run in the
sunlight, pick a dandelion
and marvel at it — what
long thoughts for a little
girl! She is so radiant and
so lovely, so full of
graceful beauty...

Let us be worthy parents, Lord, always there when our child-daughter needs us. Let us measure up to her expectations, justify her faith in us, cushion her hurts, share her joys.

Let us set an example
of love. Let her say,
when she is grown:
"Thank you for being
good parents; thank
you for being good
friends."

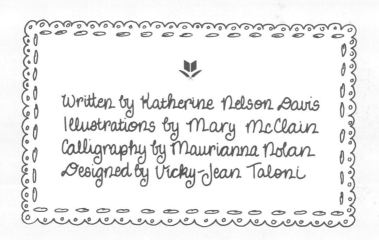

Written by Katherine Nelson Davis
Illustrations by Mary McClain
Calligraphy by Maurianna Nolan
Designed by Vicky-Jean Taloni